# Bodyweight

## Bodyweight 2.0 Workout Guide to Boosting Raw Strength and Getting Ripped Using Calisthenics, Isometrics and Cross Training

# Table of Contents

# Introduction

First of all, thank you for purchasing this book! I hope that you are able to derive a great deal of knowledge from it, as I have worked long and hard to make it as informative as possible.

I have always had a passion for strength training, and my vast experience has taught me that bodyweight training is the best way to get fit, get ripped or just work out in general.

Everything you need you already have with you; you just need to know how to use it! I created this book so that people who are wasting their time with gyms and other gimmicks can start using their own body weight instead and see just how useful a bodyweight workout can be.

In this book you are going to learn just what bodyweight training actually is. I will discuss the differences between the three branches of bodyweight training, which are calisthenics, isometrics and cross training, and also explain in detail about advanced and basic exercises.

You are also going to find an entire workout plan that you'll find extremely easy to apply to your daily routine! Additionally, this book contains several dietary tips that you can use to help supplement your workout routine. After all, just exercising is never enough; you are going to have to change your diet as well if you want to experience those high gains!

Another useful feature of this book is a list of benefits that you can derive by applying bodyweight training techniques to your daily workout. I hope this book helps you in your journey. Good luck!

# Chapter 1:
# What is Bodyweight Training?

In this modern day and age, taking care of one's health and ensuring that one's body is the best that it can be is an important part of the daily routine of the vast majority of people.

As a result, we tend to spend quite a bit of money going to gyms and using expensive machinery that is supposedly custom designed to help us become muscular and ripped.

However, what most of us don't know is that it is actually not necessary to spend so much money and waste so much time on gyms when we can just work out at home!

Working out at home is possible with bodyweight exercises. Bodyweight training essentially involves a wide variety of exercises that can be split into three basic types. These three basic types are described below:

## Calisthenics

The key to these exercises is rhythmic movement that does not require any form of specialized equipment. When one thinks of bodyweight exercises, calisthenics is what usually comes to mind.

Calisthenics is the foundation of the bodyweight training world. These exercises include pushups, squats, pull-ups, sit-ups, and all other exercises that involve repetitive and rhythmic movement.

Calisthenics is the oldest form of exercise in the world. Weight training is a relatively recent innovation. Before it was invented, soldiers would do calisthenics in order to stay fit.

Even today, the militaries of the world use calisthenics – not weight training – in order to gauge the fitness of potential soldiers, simply because it is more convenient. In fact, calisthenics is actually the origin of modern weight training. The bench press, the pull down, the leg press: all of these are simulations of actual calisthenics exercises. Why pay for the simulation when you can just do the real thing for free?

## Isometrics

Isometrics and calisthenics have one major difference: movement. Isometric exercises involve getting into a position in which the muscles are tense and staying in that position for as long as possible.

An example of this would be to go halfway up during a sit up and stay there. Your muscles will remain tense and will begin burning in no time.

Most isometric exercises can actually be used in conjunction with calisthenics in order to improve the efficacy of the calisthenics workout. In this manner, calisthenics and isometrics are intrinsically connected to one another.

## Cross training

Cross training refers to an interdisciplinary branch of exercise. This essentially involves applying practice techniques from basketball, football, swimming and various different sports in order to create a versatile workout.

This is actually quite effective, because each exercise allows you to focus on a different aspect of your physique. Cross training can also involve circuit training, which involves running between two points while a beeper times you. The goal is to reach the other end before the beeper goes off. The beeper goes off more quickly each time, forcing you to run faster and faster until you are finally unable to beat it.

Simply put, bodyweight training refers to exercise done by using only the body's weight, instead of external weights like barbells and dumbbells. In this age, when everyone is suddenly health conscious, gyms are becoming overcrowded. It's hard to find free machines or the proper weights, and it's also a hassle to find a proper gym, get there at a decent hour before the rush, complete your workout and get back to your house or office. Bodyweight training is a lifesaver in this regard. You can train in the privacy of your home, for as long or as little you want to. You get to decide how much you want to do on a particular day.

# Chapter 2:
# Benefits of Bodyweight Training

Now that you know what bodyweight training is, let's look at the reasons this exercise routine is worth your time. After all, the gym serves you well enough. What are the benefits of following a bodyweight training routine?

## No equipment

No more waiting because the hulk next to you is banging out supersets on the barbell or guarding the dumbbells with his life. Bodyweight requires only your body. That's it.

## Anytime, anyplace

This type of training can be done at home or while traveling, in hotel rooms, at the playground, on a hill, on the road. Just you and your body.

## Increased training frequency

As you get stronger naturally, you find yourself doing more reps and sets, and this ultimately gives you more strength.

## Greater neuromuscular demand

Have you ever watched gymnastics and wondered at the superhuman agility, strength and coordination? It all comes from rigorous bodyweight training on ropes and bars and rings, six to seven times a week. Continuous body training results in the brain recruiting more muscle fibers to compensate for torn fibers, giving you more strength.

# High gains in short amounts of time

A lot of so-called physical fitness experts would tell you that bodyweight training is not worth your time because it does not provide quick gains.

However, you need to realize that these people actually have vested interests in keeping you away from bodyweight exercises. After all, they make money by selling gym memberships.

No matter what they say, the fact remains that bodyweight training provides high gains in less time. Bodyweight training is actually much more efficient than weight training.

There is significant research that supports this claim. Remember, bodyweight exercises involve high intensity plyometric movements. However, these movements do not require any equipment to perform.

That means that when you're done with one exercise, you can move on to the next without having to get any other equipment ready. You'll have shorter rest times between exercises, which allows you to keep the intensity of the workout as high as possible for as long as possible.

When you are working out at a gym, you have to hop from one machine to the other. You also have to wipe down the machines after you are done using them. This means that your muscles end up cooling down between exercises.

Bodyweight exercises allow you no respite, so your workouts will be shorter and far more intense, resulting in quicker gains.

## Bodyweight exercises combine anaerobic with aerobic exercises

When you go to a gym you begin to get dependent on gym equipment. This means that when you use the bench press, you get an anaerobic chest workout. The same goes for every other piece of equipment in the gym.

However, aerobic exercise is also extremely important. These exercises will strengthen your cardiovascular system. Additionally, anaerobic exercises are not nearly as effective as cardio exercise at burning fat.

If you're only doing anaerobic exercise, you might start getting muscles that won't even be visible underneath all of that fat! This is probably why so many people who join gyms complain that they are getting fatter than they were before. They didn't get fat; their musculature just began to develop underneath their fat, which made their rotundity become more prominent.

There are several bodyweight exercises that tackle this issue. Bodyweight exercises such as burpees, Hindu squats and mountain climbers are all excellent ways to boost muscle tone in the lower body while simultaneously giving yourself an intense cardiovascular workout.

You will notice that a lot of leg exercises that use the weight of the body make great cardiovascular exercises as well. They also help a lot by boosting the strength of the core, which is an extremely important part of your body. By targeting the core, these exercises will help you to lose belly fat as well.

## It boosts your metabolism

Bodyweight exercises are so great because they are not just one-dimensional, mechanical movements that are meant to exercise a single muscle in your body. Instead, bodyweight exercises are holistic techniques whereby you can improve and enhance every part of your body. This includes your metabolism.

You now know that bodyweight exercises are useful at helping you lose weight because they provide cardiovascular exercise which is more efficient at burning unnecessary fat from the body.

Additionally, bodyweight exercises help burn fat by boosting your metabolism. Even a few minutes of bodyweight exercises will boost your metabolism over the course of the next few hours.

When your metabolism is high, your body is better able to metabolize fat and remove it from your system so you don't gain any more weight. Often, people who are predisposed to chubbiness never lose weight because they just gain back whatever they've lost due to their slow metabolism.

This concern is addressed by bodyweight exercises. These exercises prevent your body from accumulating more fat for a significant period of time after you exercise. As a result, the cardiovascular portion of your workout will end up being a lot more effective because it won't have any extra fat to burn.

This lethal combination of aerobic exercise and metabolism boosting that bodyweight exercises provide can make all of your unnecessary pounds vanish in no time, and the great thing is that you will be able to eat what you want while losing all of this weight!

## Bodyweight exercises provide an afterburn effect

You might have thought that the aerobic exercise and metabolic boost provided by bodyweight exercises were more than enough weight loss benefits, especially if you're more focused on gaining muscle.

However, bodyweight exercises also help you to lose weight in yet another way, making a trio of benefits to help you during your quest to lose the fat that is preventing your muscles from popping out and becoming prominent.

This benefit that they provide is afterburn, or excess post-exercise oxygen consumption (EPOC). Afterburn is a term used to describe a metabolic state that your body gets into after you have performed bodyweight exercises. During this afterburn, your body continues to burn fat as you are sweating, until it has cooled down to its normal temperature.

This means that even if you work out for forty-five minutes, your body will continue burning fat after your workout – for so long that it's almost like you worked out for ninety minutes instead!

This afterburn effect goes down a notch after your body has cooled down, but it does still continue to burn fat, albeit at a slightly slower rate. This truly incredibly fact about bodyweight exercises means that you can perform bodyweight exercises in the morning and the afterburn effect will have your body burning fat for the rest of the day even if you don't do anything!

# Bodyweight exercises strengthen your core

One major problem that I have with weight training is that it emphasizes the muscles that are considered to be aesthetically appealing so much that it tends to ignore muscles that actually serve a functional purpose.

One of the muscle groups that weight training tends to ignore is your core. When most people think of the core, they think of abs and claim that there are several weight-training machines that target the abs quite well.

However, the core consists of much more than just the abs. These machines tend to focus on giving you a six-pack, but just focusing on the abs without strengthening the core is very wrong. Core muscles include twenty-eight other muscles apart from the abdominals, and these muscles play important roles in digestion and posture as well.

Strengthening the core properly can allow you to relieve lower back pain and to feel better and more energetic throughout your day.

Pretty much every single bodyweight exercise that you do involves the core in some way. This is because bodyweight exercises are so natural in the way they exert your body.

The way these exercises train your core is exceptional, because they don't just build your abs. They improve your overall health as well, and can banish aches and pains that you would otherwise just have to live with.

## Bodyweight exercises keep you flexible

Another problem that I have with weight training is that the exercises involved tend to keep you stiff. Your muscles get rigid and unyielding, and spending too much time with your muscles in this state can lead to some serious damage.

Weight trainers are supposed to perform a series of stretches in order to keep their muscles supple, but most weight trainers simply ignore these stretches, thinking that they are not important. It's not even really their fault. After all, their focus is on gaining muscle, not on keeping those muscles supple.

The great thing about bodyweight exercises is that they are not nearly as stiffening as weight training exercises. Bodyweight training involves much more natural movements which force your muscles to stretch as they grow. This means that the muscles you gain will be naturally supple.

This, of course, does not mean that you will not need to stretch your muscles before and after you perform your bodyweight workout. However, you are not going to have to worry as much about stretching while performing bodyweight exercises, which is a stark contrast to weight training, where not stretching can cause serious injury if it goes on for long.

Do yourself a favor and opt for bodyweight training rather than weight training. Keep your muscles supple throughout your workout rather than making stretching a supplement to a workout that is already time consuming and tiring.

## It leaves you with no excuses not to work out

If there is one problem – or excuse, rather – that is endemic to pretty much everybody who wants to lose weight it is that they can't find the time.

If you ever ask someone who is overweight or wants to get muscular what's keeping them from simply working out and getting the job done, they will probably say that they simply don't have the time to go all the way to the gym and spend hours there working out when they have so much work that they need to do.

The great thing about bodyweight exercises is that they are completely hassle-free. They usually don't take too much time to complete, are incredibly effective, and the vast majority of them require absolutely no equipment whatsoever.

People whose training regimen involves a great deal of bodyweight training will have absolutely no excuse not to work out. Even if they have no car, even if they have absolutely no time during the day to go to the gym and exercise, they will surely be able to take half an hour every day to do some pushups, squats and pull-ups at home.

If you are the kind of person who frequently makes excuses and ends up not working out, you should give bodyweight training a try. You will have so much fun and will be done so quickly that you'll have no reason not to work out!

## Bodyweight training gives you better balance

You probably know by now that the main gripe that I have with weight training is that it is not at all versatile. The only thing that weight training gives you is muscles that look good, and absolutely nothing else of value.

Bodyweight training, on the other hand, is far more versatile than weight training. You already know that bodyweight training provides several different benefits for weight loss as well as muscle growth, and that these exercises improve flexibility as well.

You should also know that bodyweight training significantly improves your sense of balance. Even exercises that aren't normally focused on balance can be modified so that the amount of muscular resistance is proportional to the balance improvement effect.

This is mostly due to the fact that these bodyweight exercises consist of functional movements instead of mechanical movements. These movements are similar to those you use in real life, which means that your sense of balance is naturally involved when you accomplish them successfully.

You can modify the exercises to provide an even more potent boost in the balance department. For example, you can modify the squat by doing it on one leg. This requires a great amount of balance, and your body will have to improve itself in order to do it.

## Bodyweight exercises are a lot more fun to do

Weight training exercises are often incredibly restrictive. If you want to work your chest you do the bench press or a machine that targets the pectoral muscle.

If you want to target your lats, you use the pull down machine. The leg press is often used in order to train the leg muscles.

However, there is no variety. You do the same old exercises every single time as long as you keep working out.

A huge problem with this is that people tend to get bored. We simply do not function well with repetitive mechanical movements. The boring nature of weight training is probably why many people give it up so quickly. They just can't bring themselves to become robots for two hours a day anymore.

Bodyweight training is excellent in this regard. Bodyweight workouts can never be boring because there are so many different variations of every single bodyweight exercise!

There are hundreds of different kinds of pushups. The diamond pushup, the vacuum pushup, the Hindu pushup, the dive-bomber, the clap pushup. Not to mention the fact that each of these different kinds of pushups can be done with one hand to add even more variety to the mix.

With weight training, incorporating so much variety would require a truly gigantic gym. However, if you want to incorporate a little variety into your bodyweight training routines, all you have to do is use a little imagination. You might end up having a completely new workout every single day!

## You can perform bodyweight exercises anywhere

One of the restrictive aspects of weight training is that it must be performed in a gym, usually indoors. This tends to get boring, and a lot of people prefer working out outdoors where there is fresh air to breathe and the pleasant smells of nature instead of the stink of stale sweat.

Outdoor gyms are extremely rare and usually very expensive because the equipment either has to be shifted in and out, which requires quite a bit of manpower, or requires significant maintenance in order to prevent it from getting spoiled by the elements.

Creating a gym in your own home would be possible if you are filthy rich, but chances are that this is not the case.

Bodyweight exercises are so useful because you can do them anywhere you want. You can do them in your bedroom, at the gym, on your balcony, on your roof, in the park, absolutely anywhere you want to.

All you need is about four by six feet of empty space and you can perform an entire workout that touches every single part of your body without having to worry about a single piece of equipment.

## Bodyweight training doesn't cost anything

Apart from a lack of time, another very common excuse that people give for not working out is that they do not have enough money. And who can blame them?

Gyms and fitness clubs are extremely expensive. Often the upfront membership fees are not that high in order to give prospective gym goers the feeling that it's affordable, but the tiny surcharges that you incur without even realizing it, by stepping into the pool, using the sauna, using a particular piece of equipment, add up to make the whole thing far too expensive.

This is what makes bodyweight training great. If you genuinely don't have enough money to go to the gym, you don't have to!

Just apply bodyweight training techniques at home and you won't have to spend a single penny on getting the ripped muscles that you have always wanted.

In fact, the recent rise in popularity of bodyweight training is probably connected to the fact that working out in your own home costs absolutely nothing, whereas going to the gym is both time consuming and prohibitively expensive for the average person.

## Bodyweight training is less likely to cause injury

It is a common enough story that you have probably heard before. The aspiring body builder's heart burst, or his muscle ruptured, or he sprained a joint or broke a bone because he was so eager to get ripped.

However, doesn't it seem odd to you that going to the gym, which is supposed to be good for you, can be so dangerous? On the other hand, bodyweight training has never been connected to such injuries. The reason is that bodyweight training is simply not as dangerous as regular weight training.

Remember that bodyweight exercises are natural movements. They do not put additional pressure on your body because the weight you are using is that of your body itself. Your body is always handling its own weight, which means that when you use this weight in order to exercise your joints are far more able to take the strain.

This contrasts drastically with weight training, where gym goers often lift weights that are far too heavy for them and get injured as a result. Even people who don't get injured end up developing aches and pains that plague them for the rest of their lives.

These aches and pains are one of the biggest reasons why people are afraid of working out. Bodyweight training is so safe that it's often used to rehabilitate people.

If you're afraid of getting injured, or are already injured and don't want to exacerbate your injury by going to the gym, give bodyweight exercises a shot. You will find that these exercises are stimulating, effective, and do not put any unnecessary or injury-inducing strain on your body.

## Bodyweight training provides better results

Bodyweight training is more efficient than weight training because you don't have to rest between each exercise while you prep the next machine or piece of equipment for the next step in your workout.

However, bodyweight training is also more effective than weigh training because of a fundamental difference between these styles of exercise.

Weight training focuses almost entirely on isolation exercises. This means that the exercises that are performed during weight training target specific muscles and none of the outlying or surrounding muscles.

This may seem useful, because you are not wasting energy on muscles that you don't need, but the truth is that isolating one muscle while avoiding another is actually terrible for your body. You will end up developing muscles in a disproportionate manner, because it is simply impossible to apply the exact same amount of strain to each isolated muscle in your body.

This isolation-based training also ignores tiny supportive muscles. This means that you might develop bulging biceps, but these biceps won't be as strong as they look because their support muscles (which help them to lift things) won't be as strong as they are.

This is where bodyweight training is fundamentally different from weight training. Bodyweight exercises are called compound exercises because they target several different muscles at the same time.

For example, pushups target your chest, shoulder and triceps muscles. They also strengthen your hands along with the muscles along your rib cage. This means that each muscle will develop proportionately, and your muscular chest and shoulders will be a lot more functionally useful.

In essence, doing pushups gives you the same definition in your chest muscles as the bench press, but it makes your chest muscles a lot stronger.

## Incidental training

What happens when you bench press? You obviously hit your chest, deltoids and triceps. Now try a one-hand pushup. Felt the difference? Apart from your pecs, deltoids and triceps, your lats have come into the picture to protect your shoulders, your abs and glutes remain tight to keep your hips from sagging, and your quads and hamstrings stretch to keep the legs straight. Full body movement. This is incidental training.

# Chapter 3:
# Understanding Your Body

Before we delve into the different exercises you can perform, let's look at what you must keep in your mind when you are trying to build muscle through a body weight routine.

## What to keep in mind

### Low reps

This is the only strategy that will work. Keep your reps low in number. Doing pushups for an hour will not give you a huge chest.

### Go to fatigue

You need to push yourself and be straining at the last rep, gasping for breath. Otherwise you will not make any changes to your body. The last few reps should be extremely demanding. You should literally collapse at the end.

### Circuits

Try to get as many circuits as possible in your time frame. For example, if you have only 20 minutes for your workout, make sure to include compound movements like squats, lunges, pull-ups, pushups, squat jumps, burpees and planks to give you a total body workout.

### Warming up and cooling down

Not being in the gym doesn't mean you don't warm up or cool down. Exercising without warming up will only harm you in the long run. If your muscles are not warm enough for exercise, you will injure yourself as you try the more advanced moves. Cooling down is equally important. The muscles have been stretched beyond their capacity. You need to cool them down with some dynamic stretching.

The only disadvantage with bodyweight training is the lack of progressive overload. For a muscle to grow, it needs continuous overloading. In the gym, it is possible to break the muscle fibers with steadily increasing weights. Once the muscle fiber breaks down, it gets repaired while resting and grows back bigger and stronger. The next progressive overload breaks it down again and it grows back again. So on and so forth.

In bodyweight training, the muscle mass increases at first, but as it gets used to the body's weight, there is no further breakdown of the fibers and therefore no growth. One way to combat this is to keep increasing the time under tension. The more time a muscle fiber is under tension, the more the resistance and the more it breaks.

Now that we have the basics out of the way, let's get started with some basic bodyweight exercises.

## Body parts to focus on

There are several different exercises that you can begin incorporating into your workouts. However, it is very important to partition them into three different categories.

These categories are exercises that target the upper body, midsection and lower body.

### Upper body

Exercises that target the upper body essentially target the chest, shoulders, arms and upper back.

This area is so diverse, with so many different muscles, that we are going to have to include two basic exercises in this section.

The first exercise is obviously the pushup. The pushup is the king of calisthenics, and is probably the first ever exercise that was ever invented.

Before the pushup, exercise essentially involved running around or performing activities specific to your job, such as performing drills in the military. The pushup was the first exercise specifically intended to build muscle mass and improve overall strength.

In order to do a pushup, first lie in a prone position, facing the floor and supporting your body with your hands spread out and your elbows locked.

Form is very important, so you need to make sure that your arms are a little wider than shoulder length apart and that your back is completely straight.

This means that your backside should not be sticking out, nor should it be curving inwards. Doing pushups with improper posture could cause serious injury, so make sure you use proper form for this exercise.

Once your form is perfect, lower your upper body to the ground by bending your arms at the shoulders. You should keep descending until your nose is almost touching the ground and then push yourself back up.

It is absolutely essential that you keep your back completely straight while you are doing pushups so you don't develop abnormal muscles.

If you find pushups too difficult to do this way, try doing them on your knees instead of on your feet. This will help you by giving you less weight to push back up, allowing you to build up strength until you are able to do regular pushups properly.

The other upper body exercise that you can perform is the pull-up. Pushups target your chest, shoulders and triceps. Pull-ups, on the other hand, target your upper back, your rear shoulders and your biceps. Doing both these exercises will give you a more balanced musculature than doing just one.

In order to do a pull-up you need to find some sort of sturdy metal rod that you can hang from with all of your body weight. Once you are hanging, leave your entire body loose and pull yourself up using just your upper back.

Make sure you don't twist around while going up, which could cause injury. Your palms can face you, which makes the pull-ups easier and puts more focus on your biceps, or you can have them facing away from you. This will make the pull-ups more difficult to do and put more of the focus on your upper back.

If you can't do any pull-ups, trying hanging from the rod for a period of time. This will strengthen your back until you are able to do pull-ups.

### Midsection

This is another extremely important part of your body that you will need to tackle. For this section, there's just one exercise that targets your entire abdominal area.

Your abs can be the most attractive muscles in your entire body. In order to develop them, you need to do sit-ups.

Sit-ups are quite easy to do. You simply lie on your back, tuck your knees in and raise your upper body until it touches your knees, then descend back down.

It is recommended that you keep your hands crossed in front of you rather than keeping them behind your neck. This is because if you keep your hands behind your neck, you might end up using the strength of your arms rather than your abdominals.

Additionally, try to ensure that you do not twist around while raising your body. Your body should rise in a straight arc and settle back down the same way. You should also consciously attempt to raise yourself up using your abdominal muscles rather than any other muscle in your body.

It is often quite hard to do sit-ups correctly, so if you feel they are too difficult, do crunches instead. Crunches are half the motion. You raise your upper body high enough to flex your abs and then go back down. Doing crunches can help strengthen your body for sit-ups.

### Lower body

Skipping leg day is a problem endemic to people who work out. Leg muscles are often ignored because they do not provide much aesthetic value. However, ignoring them can result in a disproportionate body that is certainly not attractive.

The best exercise for your lower body is squats. Squats can be performed by standing with your feet shoulder width apart, squatting down and then getting back up again. This exercise is excellent for developing your thighs and glutes.

However, if you really want to exercise your calves you should do calf raises. These just involve standing in the same position as for squats, standing on your tiptoes, and then descending back down.

This exercise will really burn your calves and get some definition in there, and will also provide a more direct workout to your glutes.

Using these two exercises you can give your lower body a comprehensive workout.

# Chapter 4:
# Exercises for the Chest

You might think that a loaded barbell or a set of heavy dumbbells are the only way to build a strong, muscular chest. Wrong. You can develop an impressive set of pecs just by using your own body and arms, without lifting a single piece of equipment at the gym. There is a simple three-phase setup for doing this. The first phase builds your endurance levels, the second one boosts your strength, and the third one packs in the explosiveness needed for you to add size and bulk to your chest. And what's more, all you need to do are some variations of the standard pushup. Yes, it's that simple. And that difficult.

Let's first figure out some key points in chest building. Your chest is made up of four major muscle groups, namely, the pectoralis major, the pectoralis minor, the subclavius and the serratus anterior. In order to get the optimum results, all of these muscle groups need to be worked on. While weight training, one has the advantage of progressively overloading the muscles every week or with each set. With bodyweight training, however, the key focus should be on the time each muscle group is kept under tension. Since the muscle fibers cannot be overloaded week after week, the time under tension will provide the resistance necessary to build the muscle. The human body does not know whether the resistance is from a barbell or a dumbbell or a cable or its own weight. All it knows is that something is pushing it or it has to pull something. Of course, as with every exercise, proper form is of utmost importance. You need to hit the full range of motion in every single rep. Cheating and poor form will get you nowhere.

Always aim to get at least 5-7 reps on each set. It will get better as you get stronger.

# The pushup and its variations

The pushup is simply one of the best bodyweight exercises. It's not just good for the chest, but the core and arms as well. In a regular pushup, one gets into the pushup position on all fours, back straight, arms just below the shoulders, and lowers the body to the ground in a straight line until the chin almost touches the floor and then back up. Let's look at some variations of the pushup:

### Incline pushup

People who have trouble doing the basic pushup can start with this. This exercise targets the main chest muscles but puts less pressure on the elbows and also considerably reduces the amount of body weight that is being lifted. Incline pushups can be done against any solid surface, such as a desk, a wall, a tabletop etc.

- Face the surface (table, desk or wall) and place your arms on it, slightly wider than shoulder width.

- With your body in a straight line, bend forward until your face is close to the surface. Make sure your back is rigid all this time. Go back to the starting position.

### Decline pushup

This is slightly harder than an incline pushup. Your feet are elevated and you need to exert more force in your arms to lift your body.

- Choose an elevated surface, like a chair, bed or bench. Make sure it's not too high for you.

- Place your feet on the surface with your hands below your shoulders and your entire body in one straight line.

- Lower your body until your hands are perpendicular to your shoulders. Do not let your hips sag or your back bend. Quickly lift your body to its earlier position.

### Wide hand pushup

The hands are placed slightly wider apart than with a normal pushup. The movement is the same, but this variation targets your biceps as well as your pecs.

### Diamond pushup

Nothing beats this exercise when it comes to sculpting a great-looking chest. Plus, it targets your triceps as well.

- Get in the pushup position. Form a diamond with your hands and place them beneath your shoulders.

- Keeping your abs, glutes and back tight and straight, lower yourself to the floor and keep your elbows close to your body.

- Lift yourself up the same way.

### Cross over box pushup

This one is great for building your strength as well as your chest. You need an object like a sturdy box or a plate that can be fixed at one point.

- Adopt a pushup position, with one hand on the box or plate.

- Lower yourself, and while lifting your body back up, switch your hands explosively, so that the other one lands on the object. That's one rep.

- Alternate hands while lifting yourself up.

## Spiderman Pushup

- Get into a normal pushup position.

- As you lower your body, bring your right knee up to your right elbow. Keep it like this till you lift yourself up.

- On the next rep, bring your left leg to your left elbow. Continue for as many reps as you can do without losing form.

## The Hindu pushup

- Get into the pushup position.

- Raise your hips high.

- When lowering yourself, instead of going in a straight line, arch your back and dive slightly, with your head and hips sticking out.

- Lower yourself until your chest reaches the ground, then lower your hips and hold the position for a few seconds. Repeat.

# Chapter 5:
# Exercises for the Shoulders

Now that you have a drool-worthy chest, it's time to work the shoulders. In order to get well-sculpted shoulders, you need to hit all the muscles that make them up. These are the deltoids, the rotator cuff group, trapezius, serratus anterior, subclavius and pectoralis minor.

Given below are some bodyweight shoulder exercises, ranging from easy to hard. Take it easy and do not jump headfirst into the hardest exercise. You might get frustrated and give up, or hurt yourself. Don't dismiss these shoulder exercises as being too mundane; possessing strong shoulders also gives you overall strength.

In order to pack some muscle onto your shoulders, keep the rep range low, between 6-10, and also increase the time under tension. In bodyweight training, this is the only resistance that can be offered to the body. Try the following exercises carefully and with proper form.

## Single arm plank

- Get down on all fours. Straighten your legs and your core.

- Lower your hands till your elbows form a ninety-degree angle with your shoulders. Keep them beneath your shoulders. This is your standard plank position.

- Now, extend your right hand forward, as if reaching for something, keeping the rest of your body in a straight line. Hold for a few seconds.

- Return the hand to its original position and extend the left hand forward.

## Crab walk

This is a great exercise for shoulder strength. It uses the stabilizer muscles and the deltoids. Try walking backwards, if you need a challenge!

- Sit with your hands behind your shoulders.

- Slowly lift your hips, letting your glutes hang in the air, with your knees bent.

- Walk forward, with your right leg and left arm, then your left leg and right arm.

- Brace your shoulders and keep them tight. Repeat as many rounds as you can.

## Planche pushup

This is an awesome gymnastics skill exercise in which the body is held parallel to the ground, supported by the arms and shoulders. It requires great strength and balance. To make it slightly easier, a pushup version of the planche is given below.

- Get down on the floor, in a normal pushup position.

- Instead of placing your hands directly below your shoulders, make a ninety-degree angle with your waist. Your palms should be at the sides of your waist, the elbows in a straight line with your back. Think of the chaturanga pose in yoga.

- Keeping the body straight, lift yourself up, hold for a few seconds, and then lower the body till it is parallel to the floor. This is one rep. Do as many as possible without losing form.

## Elevated pike pushup

- Get into a normal pushup position.

- Keep your feet on an elevated surface, such as a table, bed or bench.

- Bend your hips, raising your hips and butt towards the ceiling, so that your torso is vertical.

- Lower yourself to the floor until your head is between your hands. Get back up explosively.

# Chapter 6:
# Exercises for the Back

All the time, we see gym goers focus mostly on their biceps, abs and chest. A lot of people who exercise at home also concentrate on legs, abs and arms. The back is one of the most neglected body parts, when it should occupy the first place. Why, you ask? Read on.

## Why you should work on your back

There are a few reasons why it is essential that you work on your back.

- The back contains some of the biggest and strongest muscles in the body, second only to the legs. The main muscles of the back are the trapezius, latissimus dorsi, levator scapulae and the rhomboids. If you work on your back muscles, you will gain a lot of strength and power.

- A wide, chiseled back also creates the illusion of a trimmer abdomen.

- Since most of the back exercises are compound movements, involving multiple joints and muscle groups, you will burn more calories per exercise.

- A stronger back will aid in many other exercises, like squats, deadlifts, clean and press, barbell rows etc.

The best exercises for building a strong back can be divided into three categories – muscular endurance, strength, and building muscle mass. Let's look at each of them separately.

## Muscular endurance

This basically means the ability of the muscle fibers to withstand the pressure and resistance of the exercise over a long period of time or a large number of reps per set.

### *Horizontal/vertical pull-up*

Instead of a normal pull-up, a beginner can start with either horizontal or vertical pull-ups.

- To do a horizontal pull-up (or inverted row), get under a bar or a sturdy table.

- Grab the bar with both hands, palms facing away from you. Keeping your body in a straight line, pull yourself up till your chin reaches the bar. Lower your body in a line.

- For a vertical version, you may use door handles or a towel wrapped around a vertical structure. Grab the handles or the ends of the towel. Keep your body straight and pull yourself towards the door. Get back into position without letting your back hunch.

### *Squat pull-up*

- You will need a bar for this.

- Squat on the floor, making sure your knees are in line with your toes.

- When you get back up, immediately grab the bar and pull yourself up. This is one rep.

# Strength

For developing strength, your exercises should be in the 6-8-rep range.

### One arm pull-up

The name itself strikes fear among even elite gym goers. Mastering pull-ups will get easier with time, but one arm pull-ups are surely a test of your arm and back strength.

- Get in a basic pull-up position, arms hanging straight from the bar.

- Bring one hand down to your side and use only one hand to pull yourself up completely.

### Tuck front lever pull-up

The front lever is one of the toughest exercises for building a strong back. It is a gymnastic move, and most people are not able to do even the back lever, a relatively easy version, even after months of practice. A simpler variation of this is the tuck front lever.

- Grasp the bar with an overhand grip.

- Lean back and pull your legs and hips up, forming a curve with your lower body. Your back should be rounded and the legs and knees tucked as tightly as possible.

- Now, try to pull yourself up slowly. Get back to the original position.

# Building muscle mass

### *The pull-up*

This old time favorite is still a hot commodity as far as building back mass goes. It is definitely one of the best exercises for a wide back and shapely lats.

- Grab hold of a bar and hang all the way down. Your arms should be straight. The grip should be slightly wider than your shoulders.

- Pull yourself up until your chin is above the bar. Your back may form a slant at this point, but that's all right.

- Lower yourself all the way down.

- Do not swing your body for the momentum. All the work has to be done by your arms and back muscles.

### *Isometric pull-up holds*

This is done in three phases.

- Pull yourself up in a normal pull-up position and hold it for 30-45 seconds.

- Lower yourself down, hanging straight, and rest for 30 seconds. Then pull yourself up so that your elbows are bent at 90 degrees. Hold for 15 seconds. Lower yourself and rest for 30 seconds.

- From a dead hang, pull yourself up only 2 inches and hold for 15-20 seconds. This constitutes one rep.

# Chapter 7:
# Exercises for Your Abdomen or Core

The abdominal muscles (or abs) are perhaps the most worked-on body part. Whether it be at a gym or within the comfort of their homes, people everywhere are obsessed with getting a flat, toned tummy. While the male population hankers after six-packs, women are preoccupied with getting a bikini-ready body.

In order for the abs to show, a man's body fat levels should be at 6-8%, while a woman's should be at 12-13%. When the core muscles become stronger and show definition, it will burn the abdominal fat. A proper diet also goes a long way toward giving you results.

Forget about torturing your abs with hundreds of crunches and sit-ups. They will not banish the fat around your midsection. Instead, try the following exercises to strengthen your core and get those muscles to pop out.

## The plank

This one isometric exercise truly blasts and destroys your abs. It strengthens the whole body, builds a strong core, strengthens the back and also builds your shoulders.

- Get into a pushup position.

- Bend your elbows 90 degrees and rest your weight on your forearms. They should be directly beneath your shoulders.

- Form a straight line with your body and hold the position for as long as you can, without letting your hips sag.

## Side crunch

Along with the core, it also works the obliques.

- Kneel on the floor, place your right palm on it and lean towards your right side.

- Balance your weight, slowly extend your left leg and point your toes ahead.

- Place your left hand behind the head, making sure the elbow points towards the ceiling.

- Lift your leg to hip height as you extend your arm above your leg, palm facing forward. Lower to the starting position.

## Opposite arm and leg raise

- Get down on all fours.

- Slowly extend your right leg behind to hip height, in line with your back.

- At the same time, extend the left hand forward. Hold for a few seconds.

- Go back to the original position. Alternate the hand and the leg.

## Single leg stretch

- Lie on your back with your knees bent.

- As you inhale, pull your left knee in towards your chin, while raising your head to meet it.

- Lift your right leg about 45 degrees from the floor.

- Switch legs. Hold the position for at least 10 seconds.

## Side plank with leg lift

- Get into a basic side plank position.

- Press your bottom foot firmly on the ground and raise the top leg as high as you can, without dropping your hips.

## Flutter kicks

This is a fantastic exercise for your hip flexors as well as your abdominal muscles.

- Lie on your back with your arms at your sides.

- Extend your legs in the air, keeping them slightly bent at the knees.

- Lift your heels about five inches off the floor and make small, rapid scissor-like movements. Keep your abs contracted.

## Russian twist

Another wonderful exercise that targets the abs and obliques at once

- Sit on the ground with your knees bent. Keep your heels close to your butt.

- Lean back slightly, keeping the back straight.

- Extend your hands in the front and twist slowly to the left. Don't swing. Let the ribs and the abdominal muscles do the work. Twist to the right side. This is one rep.

# Chapter 8:
# Exercises for the Legs

Legs exercises are notorious for their ability to conjure images of heavy weights and fearsome machines. Most people think that they cannot build powerful legs without a loaded barbell or the squat or leg press machine. Well, it turns out that you can build a pair of extremely strong legs in the privacy of your home, without any machines or weights whatsoever.

The main muscles of the legs are the quadriceps, hamstrings, adductors (thighs) and tibialis anteriors (shins), while the gastrocnemius and soleus muscles make up the calves. The legs support the body's entire weight and therefore must be exercised regularly. The following exercises are compound movements, which will work almost all the muscle groups in the legs.

## Squats

Not for nothing is this called the king of all exercises. A proper bodyweight squat routine will fire up your quads and hamstrings like nobody's business.

- Keep your legs shoulder width apart, at a slight angle, facing outwards.

- Keeping your back straight, lower your body to the ground, like sitting on a chair.

- Make sure your knees do not extend over your toes. Go all the way down until the backs of your thighs are parallel to the ground. Hold for a few seconds and drive back up through the heels.

## Squat Jumps

A fantastic plyometric exercise, which not only works the legs but increases your heart rate as well.

- Get into a deep squat position.

- When you come up, jump as high as you can and slowly land on your knees.

- Go back into the squat position.

## Bulgarian Split Squats

- Place one leg on a chair or a bench and extend the other leg in front of you as far as you can without losing balance.

- Bend down, keeping the knee at a 90-degree angle and the back straight. Come back up. This is one rep.

## Walking Lunges

Another brilliant exercise that opens up your hip flexors, activates your glutes and gives you core stability.

- Extend one leg in front and keep the other leg straight.

- Bend till the knee of the forward leg is perpendicular to the floor.

- Keep your back straight and don't let the knee fall over the toe line.

- As you rise, bring the back leg to the front and bend down. Keep alternating the legs as you walk.

## Deep Side Lunges

A deeply underestimated exercise, this works wonderfully to strengthen the legs.

- Stand with your feet shoulder wide apart.

- Bend towards your right, push your hips lower and lower your body by pushing the right knee at a 90-degree angle.

- Keep the heels firmly planted on the floor and stretch as much as you can. Return to the starting position.

## Lunge Kicks

- Get into a basic lunge position.

- As you rise, bring your back leg to the front and explosively kick as high as you can.

- Take it to the back again and lower your body. This is one rep.

## Glute Kicks

- Get down on all fours.

- Keeping your back and arms straight, bring the right knee up to your chest.

- Take the whole leg back and stretch it behind you, as high as you can go.

- Bring it back to your chest. This is one rep.

# Chapter 9:
# Exercises for the Arms and Biceps

One of the most worked-on parts, biceps are a favorite amongst gym goers all around the world. When you want to look good in a T-shirt or show off your arms in a sleeveless top, toned biceps are the way to go. And exercising them also prevents arm sag, something women in particular are often unhappy with.

The major arm muscles are the biceps brachii, the coracobrachialis, brachialis and the triceps brachii. Of course, there are a million variations of biceps and triceps exercises in the gym, but the bodyweight exercises given below are all you really need for good results.

## Pushups

- Get down on all fours. If you can't do this with your full body, use the support of your knees.

- Keep your hands slightly wider than your shoulders.

- Keep your legs and back straight and lower yourself to the floor, until your chest touches the ground. Come back up explosively. This is one rep.

## Chin-ups

While pull-ups are excellent for building your back, chin-ups work your biceps.

- Grab the overhead bar with your hands, palms facing you.

- Keep a narrow distance between your hands. This helps put resistance on the muscle.

- Pull yourself up till your chin goes above the bar.

- Lower yourself completely. This is one rep.

## Diamond dips

Refer to Chapter Four for this excellent exercise which targets the triceps.

## Triceps dips

- Grab a bench or a chair with your hands, palms wider than your hips and facing away from you.

- Lower your body and extend your legs in front of you.

- Keep your elbows straight and push with your triceps. Return to the starting position.

# Chapter 10:
# Advanced Bodyweight Exercises

The basic exercises are great if you are just starting out, but once you have a little experience you might want some more advanced exercises to put a little more strain on your muscles.

These exercises are all extremely effective and can provide an even more intense workout than you could get at a gym. They are split into the three exercise categories that were mentioned in the previous chapter.

## Upper body

### Dive-bomber pushup

If you are looking for a slightly more advanced pushup, go for the dive-bomber pushup. This pushup puts a lot more strain on your muscles. It also targets a wider range of muscles, including your upper back.

In order to perform this pushup, assume the normal pushup position, then raise your backside in the air until your body has formed an inverted V. Then lower your body, curving your head upwards as you go down until your back is curved and you are able to look at the ceiling. Go back the same way.

These pushups are especially good for your shoulder and neck muscles, and are far more effective than weight-based exercises such as the bench press at developing your upper body muscles.

### Alternate handgrip pull-ups

Pull-ups are difficult enough as it is, but you might want to mix things up a little to get more excitement into your exercise routine.

If you bring your hands closer together your pull-ups are going to target the center of your upper back, which is your lower and upper trapezius muscles. However, the further apart your hands get, the more strain they end up putting on your lats (or "wings").

You can also mix up the handgrips by having one palm facing you and the other palm facing away from you. This will require your body to get a lot more of your core into the action, and will help you to develop a rock hard midsection.

### Handstand pushups

If you really want an extreme pushup that will give you a killer shoulder and upper back workout, you can't go wrong with the handstand pushup.

The handstand pushup is one of the most difficult pushups to do, so make sure that your physical strength is sufficient; otherwise, you might end up hurting yourself.

In order to do a handstand pushup, you will obviously have to do a handstand first. You can rest your feet against a wall in order to support yourself. Then all you have to do is lower your body and raise it using the strength of your arms.

If you want to build your strength up so you can do handstand pushups, try doing just handstands first. Stay in the handstand position for thirty seconds three times a day, and soon you will be strong enough to do handstand pushups with ease.

# Midsection

## Leg raises

If there is one problem with sit-ups, it is that they tend to favor the upper abs more than the entire abdominal area. In order to get a more well-rounded abdominal section you can do leg raises.

In order to do leg raises, simply lie straight and raise your legs, keeping them completely straight, until you form an L shape with your body. Then slowly take them back down. Try not to just drop them down, as this will only be half as effective as if you take them down slowly.

## V-ups

If you want to target your entire abdominal area at once you'll need some more advanced abdominal exercises.

V-ups are a great way to get a well-rounded abdominal section in one go. In order to do V-ups, lie flat on your back and raise both your upper body and lower body at the same time. Your fingers should touch your toes, and your body should come together like the two lines in the V meeting.

This move is very advanced, so make sure you can do a large number of sit-ups and leg raises before you attempt it.

## Coffin crunches

If you are unable to do V-ups just yet, you can give coffin crunches a shot. Coffin crunches involve you lying flat on your back and raising your upper body and lower body at the same time, except your knees must be bent instead of locked.

This is a lot easier because raising your legs up in this manner puts less strain on your lower abs. This can even result in more even abdominal muscle development, and can certainly help you build up the strength to do V-ups.

## Lower body

### *Hindu squats*

Hindu squats are an absolutely brilliant modification of the traditional squat. They are so effective because they offer significant aerobic exercise along with a much more intense leg workout. If you want tree trunk legs, your best bet is Hindu squats!

Hindu squats are a lot more rhythmic and explosive than regular squats. They involve you stretching your arms out in front of you as your legs are spread shoulder width apart and inhaling. After this, you swing your arms back as you squat down on your toes and exhale forcefully as you lunge back up.

This exercise is extremely effective. If you feel the burn and can't do more than a few, just keep in mind that the Indian wrestlers of old used to do hundreds of these every single day!

Hindu squats are the perfect leg exercise. They target your thighs, calves and glutes and offer an excellent cardiovascular workout as well. Doing these for about fifteen minutes a day can really boost your health and give your legs some well-defined musculature.

# Chapter 11:
# Bodyweight Training

## For strength

Now that we've seen some basic exercises for working the upper and lower body, as well as the core and abs, let's find out how bodyweight training can be used for building overall strength. You don't need to spend hundreds of dollars on gym memberships for this. Your own body will do the trick.

People who begin bodyweight workouts notice that for the first few months everything is working out nicely. They are gaining muscle mass and their strength is improving. All of a sudden, they notice diminishing returns. No more mass is gained; neither is strength. This is a natural progression. Most bodyweight exercises focus on the high weight, low rep principle. While this is perfectly fine at the gym, where you can gradually and steadily increase the number of pounds you lift, it gets into a plateau mode when you're doing a bodyweight workout. For example, you might have found it very difficult to do a pull-up at the beginning of your bodyweight regime. But with regular practice, you may now find it very easy to do 20 pull-ups. This means you've left the "strength" part of the continuum, and are now in the "endurance" part of it. There is no overload on your muscles now, and this is the reason for the diminishing returns.

Having said that, it is still possible to build larger and stronger muscles through a bodyweight training program. You just have to steadily increase the muscle time under tension with each set.

For a beginner strength program, keep the following points in mind:

1. Aim to do your sets in the 6-10 rep range for everything except ab exercises, which can be done in the 20-25 rep range.

2. Keep a workout record to keep track of what you've been doing.

3. Keep your resting time between sets to a minimum, between 45-60 seconds.

4. Train for 4-5 days a week and take 1-2 days completely off.

### A beginning strength program

I'm giving you a basic bodyweight circuit here. A circuit routine means that each of the exercises will be done in succession, without any breaks. A rest period of 1-2 minutes is allowed at the end of the circuit. Go for as many rounds as possible without losing form on any of the exercises. If you feel you are slipping, take a break, catch your breath and continue.

Always warm up before you begin. A good warmup makes sure that your heart is pumping and your muscles and joints are all warmed up. You may do either static or a dynamic warmup, as given below:

- Wrist rotations – 10, each wrist

- Elbow rotations – 10, each elbow, each side

- Hand rotations – 10, each hand, each side

- Side bends – 10, each side

- Windmills – 10, each side

- Foot rotations – 10, each foot

- Jogging in place – 30 seconds

After the warmup, start the workout as follows:

- 20 bodyweight squats

- 10 pushups

- 20 walking lunges

- 10 triceps dips

- Pull-ups – as many as possible

- 15-second plank

- 30 jumping jacks or jumping in place or skipping rope

Do this circuit as many times as possible. Make sure to stretch properly afterwards. Your muscles have been contracted during the pushing and pulling movements, so give them a nice stretch. Do this routine 2-3 times a week, but not on consecutive days. Your body needs to recover from the workout. You don't build muscle when you're exercising; you build it when you rest. Do not work on the same muscle groups two days in a row. Give at least 48 hours for the muscle group to recover.

Along with workouts, a proper diet goes a long way in ensuring your health and gains. Just because you did an intense bodyweight session does not mean you can binge on pizza or burgers or fries. Eat natural, fresh products from the farm, cook nutritious meals at home, eat lots of fruits and vegetables, and drink gallons of water.

## For fat loss – high intensity interval training (HIIT)

HIIT, or high-intensity interval training, or Tabata training is doing an exercise for a given period of time at full intensity, and then taking a micro-break of a few seconds before continuing the next set. It is basically a series of quick, intense bursts of exercise, with very short recovery periods. The greatest advantage of this technique is that your heart rate speeds up quickly and you burn more fat in less time. You may feel your muscles begin to strain and feel like they're on fire. This is nothing but the beginning of our old friend afterburn or EPOC. During the EPOC stage, the anaerobic system takes over. During exercise, the phosphate in the blood is used up first, and then lactic acid and glycolysis come into play, giving you the "burn" in your muscles. Any sort of intense exercise definitely gets your metabolism running in high gear and helps you burn more fat. Some benefits of HIIT are:

1.  It increases your metabolic rate. That means that your body will continue burning calories long after you've stopped exercising, in order to replenish all the lost oxygen. This afterburn effect continues up to 48 hours after your workout. You might just be sitting still, but you'll still be burning calories.

2.  Less time is wasted with HIIT workouts, which only require 20-25 minutes. These workouts can be done anywhere, anytime. If you're hard pressed for time, or have only 20-30 minutes every other day, this is perfect for you.

3. It does not require the use of any equipment like dumbbells or barbells or kettle bells. HIIT mainly uses body weight and focuses primarily on increased heart rate and optimum muscle building.

This intense burst of activity stimulates the muscle-building hormones, such as the growth hormone and IGF-1. This, in turn, prepares your body to shed its fat and build lean mass. The shorter resting time between sets ensures that your cardiovascular health is also improved, making you recover faster in future workouts.

HIIT places a lot of stress on your body. It needs time to heal after the workout, so do not do HIIT more than thrice a week. On alternate days or rest days you can do some light cardio or strength training, but also make sure that you keep one day completely off from any sort of training. As I said before, muscles are built not while exercising, but while resting.

All right then, gear up! Get ready to blast your body through an amazing workout, which will have far greater returns than you can imagine now. Perform each exercise for 20 seconds, going all out. Then rest for 10 seconds. Exercise for 20 seconds, rest 10 seconds. Complete eight rounds of each exercise. Rest for one minute before going on to the next one.

### A basic HIIT workout

Your warmup can be static or dynamic, although a dynamic warmup is better. Jog in place for 30 seconds, do 30 jumping jacks and jump rope for 30 seconds.

- Bodyweight squats

- Pushups

- Sit-ups

- Jump squats

- Triceps dips

- 30-second burpees

I've already explained how to do bodyweight squats, push-ups, jump squats and tricep dips.

For sit-ups, lie down on your back, with your knees bent. Keeping your core tight, raise your head and back off the ground, towards your chest, until your back is at a 90-degree angle to the floor. Hold for a few seconds and get back to the starting position.

For burpees, get into a squat position. Squat till your hips are almost parallel to the ground. Bring your hands to the front and explosively jump back, straightening your legs behind you in a pushup position. Jump back to a squat, and as you rise, jump as high as possible. Return to the squat position.

If this becomes too easy for you, try the other two workouts given below. You may also do them as a circuit. Do not rest in between sets while doing a circuit. Do as many reps as possible within 20-25 seconds.

# Chapter 12:
# The Workout

## Warmup

Start with toe touches. In order to get as much stretch as possible, stretch your fingers upwards as if you are trying to touch the ceiling and then bring your arms down to touch your toes. You will end up stretching further.

Additionally, stretch your arms by swinging them around in a windmill motion. You should also stretch your midsection by bending backwards and your sides by stretching sideways.

You should also run in place for a few minutes to get your blood flowing. This will make you more energetic while doing these exercises.

## Beginner's workout

### Upper body

If you are an absolute beginner, start with one set of five pushups per day. Otherwise you can start off with five sets of five. Increase the amount of pushups in each set by one per day until you are doing twenty pushups per set.

Ideally, you should do one dive-bomber per set and increase in the following manner:

1. Monday: 1×5

2. Tuesday: 2×1, 1×4

3. Wednesday: 2×2, 1×3

4. Thursday: 2×3, 1×2

5. Friday: 2×4, 1×1

6. Saturday: 2×5

You are essentially increasing one pushup per set per day until you are doing one extra pushup in each set. Keep increasing until you are doing twenty pushups per set.

Your second upper body exercise is the pull-up. You should do half as many pull-ups per set as you do dive-bomber pushups. If you are at the beginner level and unable to do pull-ups, hang from the bar for thirty seconds and try as hard as you can to pull yourself up.

Handstand pushups as well as alternate grip pull-ups can be done for the upper body but are not required if you are doing both dive-bomber pushups and standard pull-ups.

### Midsection

Your midsection exercises are V-ups, and you will do the same number of V-ups per set as dive-bombers. This means that if you are doing five sets of five dive-bombers, you will do five sets of five V-ups as well.

If you cannot do V-ups, do leg raises and sit-ups instead. The ratio should be two leg raises and two sit-ups per dive-bomber. This means that if you are doing five sets of five dive-bombers, you are going to do five sets each of ten leg raises and ten sit-ups.

Increase until you are able to do twenty V-ups per set.

### *Lower body*

The ideal exercise for the upper body is the Hindu squat. You should do five Hindu squats per set for each diver-bomber pushup that you do.

This means that if you are doing five sets of five dive-bombers, you will be doing five sets of twenty-five Hindu squats.

You can do regular squats instead of Hindu squats coupled with calf raises if you are not strong enough to do Hindu squats. These should be done at a ratio of eight per dive-bomber per set.

## Workout 1

Round One: burpees, mountain climbers, jumping jacks, jump rope for 3 minutes.

Round Two: walking lunges, reverse lunges, squats, pull-ups, plank, jump rope for 3 minutes. In reverse lunges, instead of bringing the leg to the front, bring the leading leg behind and keep the alternate leg straight.

Round Three: burpees, squats, skater's lunges, diver's pushups, jump rope for 3 minutes.

For skater's lunges, stand with your feet slightly wider than shoulder width. Bring your right foot behind the left one, as far as it can go, and bend both knees into a lunge. Keep the right foot behind the left heel. Return to the starting position and change the legs.

For diver's pushups, make an inverted "V" shape with your body, your hands straight, your legs stretched out behind and your hips in the air. Lower your body until your chest is almost parallel to the ground, then raise your body upwards, like a cobra. At this point, your chest should be out, your back arched, arms straight. Hold it and return to the starting position.

A slightly advanced HIIT routine is given below. Do the exercises in pairs, A and B. Do each one for 20-25 seconds, as many reps as possible, then rest for 10 seconds. Continue till you complete eight rounds of each pair.

## Workout 2

A – Star jumps

B – Clapping pushups

For star jumps, get into a squat position. As you rise, jump up explosively, but this time, extend your hands and legs as you jump, so that your body resembles the shape of a star. Land lightly on your knees and resume the squat position.

In clapping pushups, as you lift your body up from the floor, bring both your hands together very quickly and place them back in position as you get ready to lower yourself down.

A – Squat jumps

B – Crunches

A – Jumping lunges

B –Back bow crossovers

For the crossovers, lie on your stomach. Slowly extend your hands in front of you as if reaching for something.

Simultaneously, lift your legs from the ground as high as they can go, so that your whole body is supported on your stomach.

A – Double burpees

B –Hindu pushups

For double burpees, stand with your feet hip-width apart, squat down and place your hands in front of your body. Kick back explosively and do two pushups. Come back to the starting position, do two back lunges and stand again. This is one rep.

Plank – for 60 seconds

# Chapter 13:
# The Accompanying Diet

Everywhere you look, in the papers, on the net, in TV advertisements, each day brings a new diet plan guaranteed to make your fat disappear and give you gleaming six-pack abs, all by summer. There are so many myths surrounding this particular aspect of health, it's staggering. Here are a few of them. I'm sure you've come across them at some point in your life.

- Chocolate gives you acne.

- Eating carbs after 7 pm makes you fat.

- The healthiest diet to follow is low-fat, low-carb, high-protein with lots of grains.

- Eat several small meals a day, instead of three large meals.

- Avoid eating egg yolks.

- Eating fat makes you fat.

- Refrain from eating dairy products, as they are full of fat and unwanted calories.

- Sugar causes diabetes.

- Fasting in the morning can help you lose weight.

Whew! These are only some of the myths that keep doing the rounds of the internet and papers. People fall headlong for such untested and unscientific statements made by people who haven't the faintest clue what they're harking on about. What a lot of people fail to understand is that the diet is a very important part of the whole workout regimen. Here are a few tips that will help you make the progress you want.

## Count calories

This may seem obvious, but you'd be surprised at how many people don't think that counting your calories is important.

Remember, your muscles won't be visible if you have large quantities of fat covering them, so you need to get rid of at least some of that fat so that the fruits of your labor are there for everyone to see.

The best way to lose weight is to eat fewer calories than you are burning. This helps you lose weight because your body burns fat to get enough energy to support the exercise you're doing.

Just calculate three numbers: how many calories you need to consume to lose weight, how many calories you burn while exercising, and how many calories you eat each day. The number you eat minus the number you burn should be within your caloric intake limit.

## Boost your metabolism through your diet

Now you need to make another calculation, of the minimum number of calories that your body can process each day before it begins to convert the sugar that your food is broken down into to fat. You can do this with an online calculator or visit your doctor and get him to explain it.

After you have determined the minimum caloric intake that you can metabolize, eat no more than five hundred calories per day beyond this minimum intake. You must also make sure that you do not eat below the minimum.

Staying within five hundred calories above this minimum level will help to keep your metabolism high. If you eat more than five hundred calories above this limit your body will become sluggish and unable to digest food as fast as it should. As a result, your metabolism will slow down. Likewise, if you eat less, your body will go into starvation mode and your metabolism will drop.

## Log your calories

Many people think that once they know how many calories they're supposed to eat it will be easy to estimate how many they're consuming and stay within the limit. However, it's much more accurate to write down everything you eat. Log each food you eat and how many calories it contains so that you know exactly how much you are eating and whether you need to cut down.

This is important because we usually only count our main meals in our estimations of daily caloric intake. However, if you log every bit of food that you actually eat, you will likely find that you are sneaking in far too many calories between meals. Keeping a food log helps to avoid these between-meal snacks.

## Don't avoid fat

A common misconception among dieters is that fat must be avoided like the plague. After all, you are trying to stop being fat, so shouldn't you avoid the food that shares the name?

There are actually several different kinds of fat. It is true that you must avoid *bad* fat, which means no butter or bacon or burgers, but you should attempt to eat as much good fat as possible.

Examples of good fat are olive oil and fish. Olive oil is an excellent source of fat because it is so light, and fatty fish contains omega-3 fatty acids that your body needs.

The reason you should not cut fat out altogether is that fat is an important part of what keeps your body running. Your body actually needs fat in order to survive.

Cutting fat out completely may make you lose weight very quickly, but your health will suffer greatly as a result, and this is not a fair trade at all.

## Change your meal schedule

This is possibly one of the most important dietary tips. Your meal schedule right now probably consists of three square meals a day.

This is a fine, traditional system for most people, but it is not that conducive to weight loss. This is because your metabolism remains slow when you eat big meals that aren't metabolized properly. Your metabolism speeds up to take care of the sudden influx of food, but then when you don't eat again for a few hours it slows back down.

Instead of doing this, you should try to eat several small meals throughout the day. Whenever you eat a meal your metabolism will speed up in order to handle the influx of food, and since your meals will be small it will actually be able to do so.

Additionally, since you are going to be eating more meals throughout the day, your metabolism is going to stay high, resulting in you losing more weight than if you ate two or three big meals.

## Do not favor one over the other

Many people have trouble focusing on diet and exercise at the same time. If they are working out they ignore their diet, or conversely they focus too much on their diet and end up neglecting their workout regimen.

But if you want the body of your dreams you are going to need to pay attention to both of these things every day; otherwise, there's simply no point.

Your diet is more important than your workout for losing weight and burning fat. However, your diet will not help you build muscle. The only thing that can do that is your workout.

If you want the best of both worlds you are going to have to apply both concepts to your daily routine.

It may get difficult sometimes, because you will feel as though both of these things are restrictions, but the key is to not think of your diet as a job. Just make it the way you eat, and after a couple of weeks you will have forgotten what it was like to not be on this diet.

# Don't drink

This is probably one of the more difficult tips on this list. Alcohol is an important part of our culture and social lives, and it is just plain fun to drink.

However, you really need to quit drinking if you want to burn fat. To understand why, you must understand how alcohol is metabolized.

Alcohol is poisonous to your body, so your liver breaks it down into sugar. A little bit of alcohol is broken down into enormous amounts of sugar by your liver.

So much sugar can make you go hyperglycemic, so your body turns these sugars into fat. Drinking alcohol makes you far fatter than soda or fast food.

If you want your diet and workout routine to be effective you are going to have to cut alcohol out of your diet completely, at least until you have lost a significant amount of weight.

# Fill up on alternative proteins

It is pretty obvious that if you want to gain muscle mass you are going to need protein. After all, protein is what your body uses to rebuild your muscles after your workout has created micro-tears in them, making the muscles bigger and stronger so that they are able to handle the strain.

However, you should also know that meat isn't the best thing to eat if you want to burn fat. This is because meat contains large amounts of bad fat, which you should be avoiding.

It's better to eat chicken than red meat, but the smarter option would be to avoid meats altogether and go for vegetarian proteins. Beans, legumes and nuts are jam-packed with protein, containing far more protein per ounce than meat does.

The great thing is that this protein is very healthy, so you can eat as much of it as you want. This is just a suggestion; you can eat meat if you want to, but just keep in mind that doing so will make your diet less effective than it would be otherwise.

## Have cheat days

One of the most important aspects of the diet is the cheat day. Cheat days are essentially days where the rules of the diet don't apply, when you can eat whatever you want and however much of it you want to eat.

This is important because human beings generally don't function well under restrictive circumstances. We tend to enjoy our freedom, which means that if we restrict our diet for too long we are probably going to snap and end up abandoning it altogether.

Hence, it is essential that we follow the cheat day rule. Just pick out any day of the week – Sunday is a good choice because it is a day of relaxation and you won't be working out on that day either – and eat absolutely anything without worrying about the calories you are consuming.

If you are avoiding meat, make this cheat day the day that you can eat a steak or a burger. Remember, occasional indulgence helps you to stay faithful to the overall diet, and will help you lose a lot of weight in the long run.

# Eat as much soy as possible

This is related to the previous tip recommending you avoid protein that came from meats.

One of the most efficient sources of protein in the world is soy. It is very dense in protein, more dense than perhaps any other food, and it is readily available.

There are a lot of fake meat products that are actually made of soy. These meat products taste almost exactly like the real thing and contain far more protein and barely any fat!

Soy is also extremely healthy in moderate quantities. You can boost your daily protein intake by drinking soymilk, which has the added bonus of being absolutely delicious.

If you can't find it in you to give up meat, make a last-ditch effort and give soy products a shot. They may seem gross before you try them, but the truth of the matter is that soy products are actually quite delicious and the difference between soy products and the meat products they are supposed to replace is actually quite small.

## How do you make sure you stay healthy?

Almost all nutritionists agree on certain principles for keeping the body healthy and sound.

### Never skip breakfast

Even if you're hard pressed for time, have a bowl of fruit and milk. Or brown bread with peanut butter. Skipping breakfast will cause hunger pangs later in the day, and you are more likely to munch unhealthy stuff like chips or candy bars to combat the hunger. Have a hearty breakfast and watch your energy levels stay up all through the morning.

### Go easy on fast food

There's no reason to give up on your favorite pizzas, burgers, fries and tacos. Just make sure you have them in a limited quantity at fixed time intervals, say once a month. Even better, make them at home. Then you'll have total control over the ingredients and can make healthier versions.

### Eat real food

This means food grown on a farm. Whole grains, rice, wheat, maize, millet, beans, pulses, fruits, vegetables, and nuts all constitute healthy and whole food. Eating homemade meals made of these will satiate you hunger, fill you with good calories and keep your metabolism active. Anything out of a box is a no-no. Focus on raw ingredients.

### Drink, drink, drink

By that, I mean water. Drink as much as you think you need. Forget about the 8-glass rule or the 5-liter rule. Your body will tell you when it wants food and water. Drink and eat accordingly.

### Eat good fats

Eating fat won't make you fat. Nuts, butter, and avocados all contain good fats that help your joints and muscles function smoothly and don't clog your arteries. Eat them in a moderate amount.

Do not fall prey to the diet fads cropping up every day. Listen to your body; it is smarter than you think it is. Feed it good, wholesome food and exercise daily. You will remain healthy for a long time.

Your body is the only place you have to live in. Make it beautiful. Make it healthy. Start now.

# Chapter 14:
# CrossFit

According to the definition given on the official site, "CrossFit is the principal strength and conditioning program for many police academies and tactical operations teams, military special operations units, champion martial artists and hundreds of other elite and professional athletes worldwide."

In simple terms, CrossFit is a program that provides you with a set of extremely challenging and varied workouts which boost your strength and stamina. Every day, there is a new workout, called the Workout of the Day (WOD). It will test a different aspect of your functional strength. CrossFit tests the entire body's strength, not just one particular set of muscles. A CrossFit training program ensures that your body is prepared for virtually anything.

It is unlike any gym you've been to before. It's not a commercial gym per se. There are no elliptical machines, Stairmasters, weight machines, Zumba or aerobics. What's so different about it? Well, read on.

## Who should do CrossFit?

The official site says that the program "is designed for universal scalability, making it the perfect application for any committed individual regardless of experience."

What this means is the only requirement to join a CrossFit program is tenacity, dedication, resolve and commitment. Age, gender and flexibility are no bar. You'll learn it eventually.

Each day, there is a workout posted on the site. It is not custom designed for any individual. Rather, each person does the workout to the best of his or her ability. For example, if the workout specifies squats with 140 pounds on the barbell, and if you're only able to do it with the bar (45 pounds), that is your starting point. Never mind if the guy next to you is doing squats at 200 pounds per rep. If 45 pounds is what you can do right now, that's where you'll start. Also, there are provisions for exercise substitutions. If you are unable to do squats or pull-ups or lunges, a similar movement will be substituted according to your ability and flexibility. Eventually, as you get stronger, you will be able to do the workouts as prescribed on the site or given by the instructor.

## Why CrossFit?

This section will explain to you why you should try CrossFit.

1. It's a great place to start your weight training in a non-judgmental and supportive environment. No one cares if you can't lift 100 pounds on a deadlift. If you can just lift the rod with proper form, you're good to go. People who are scared to try out weights at a regular gym or who feel conscious of others watching and judging them will be able to build confidence in a CrossFit environment.

2. Some people need more encouragement and community support and ambience to start their workouts. CrossFit' s the ideal place for that. It has a tight-knit feeling to it. Members don't just pop in to show their biceps off or grunt and yell their way towards a 500-pound deadlift. They support and care

for the newbies and heartily encourage anyone who needs help.

3. Are you someone who loves to work out every single day and feel like you've lost a loved one when you don't? Well, you'll get addicted to CrossFit in no time. Though the program is structured to give a day off in between sessions, many CrossFit fanatics end up in the gym every day, and some even come in twice a day.

## Is CrossFit dangerous? Will I hurt myself?

There have been a lot of concerns and apprehensions regarding the CrossFit program. Let's check out a few facts about it.

1. In a typical CrossFit workout, there is a target to be met. You need to complete a certain number of exercises, be it strength training or bodyweight or cardio, as fast as possible in a certain amount of time. This is where your form can suffer. You might be in a hurry to complete the workout within the time limit and sacrifice form for reps. Therefore you need an experienced and certified trainer who can keep an eye on your form. This is essential as you progress onto heavy lifting with speed. If done incorrectly, it is the fastest way of injuring yourself, and you might end up with severe, long-term injuries.

2. Some CrossFit members do end up with an incredibly serious medical condition known as rhabdomyolysis. It is very rare. This occurs when people push themselves too hard all of a sudden. The muscle fibers break down and enter the kidneys, poisoning them. This condition is mostly found in ex-athletes or weightlifters who

haven't exercised for a while, then return to the gym to prove to others how much they can lift, regardless of what their body is telling them.

So yes, if you try to go too fast and do too much, it will inevitably cause a strain on your body. Go slow and go steady.

## What to expect in your first CrossFit class

So, you've signed up for your first-ever CrossFit class. Here's what will happen:

*Dynamic warmup*

This does not mean simply running on the treadmill for ten minutes. This includes movements like jumping jacks, jumping rope, burpees, squats, pushups, pull-ups etc. These types of functional movements will complement the workout you will be doing.

*Skill/strength work*

If it is a strength day, you will work on compound lifts like squats, deadlifts, bench presses, and barbell rows. If it is a skill day, you will focus on strengthening muscle groups, with exercises like pistol squats or one-hand pushups.

*WOD*

The Workout of the Day is posted on the site or given by the instructor. You need to complete a set of exercises within a limited time period. You can do that according to your level of fitness.

*Cooldown*

A series of stretches and cooling down movements, which will balance out the rigorous activity your body has just endured. Do not skip this step.

*Example of a workout*

Five pull-ups, 10 pushups, 15 squats, 20 lunges at 20 minute AMRAP (As Many Rounds As Possible in 20 minutes)

You set your times for 20 minutes and do a circuit of the exercises, without any break between the sets. As soon as you finish your lunges, go back to the pull-ups and repeat over and over again till the time limit is up.

## CrossFit for beginners

Intimidated by the regime? Wondering how and where to start? Here are some pointers for you:

This regime is based on ten crucial and principal physical qualities: cardio, endurance, stamina, strength, power, agility, flexibility, accuracy, coordination and balance. There are different exercises that test each of the qualities, and you will do them either in pairs or groups or as a whole workout. At the end of the regime, your body should be fit enough to endure anything. The exercises are grouped together as follows:

- Aerobic activity (cardio, stamina, endurance) – running, jogging, walking, swimming, jumping rope

- Gymnastics (flexibility, strength, coordination, balance) – Handstands, rope climbing, trampoline exercises, ring exercises

- Calisthenics (coordination, flexibility, strength) – functional movements like squats, lunges, sit-ups, pull-ups, pushups, crunches

- Plyometric (power and speed) – jumps, squat jumps, burpees

- Weight lifting – snatch, clean and jerk

- Powerlifting – squats, deadlift, bench press

- Bodyweight – any functional exercise

Here are some workouts to get you started. If you can do the beginner level easily, you may move on to the advanced level.

### Beginner CrossFit bodyweight workout

*Workout 1 – 10 minutes, AMRAP*

5 pull-ups, 10 pushups, 15 squats

*Workout 2 – Three rounds; 21, 15, 9 reps*

Burpees, reverse lunges, pull-ups

*Workout 3 – Three rounds, 3 minutes, 2-minute rest between rounds, AMRAP*

15 sit-ups, 15 walking lunges, 15 pushups

### Advanced CrossFit bodyweight workout

*Workout 1 – 15 minutes, AMRAP*

One-legged squats, pull-ups, dips

*Workout 2 – three rounds, 3 minutes, 1 minute rest between rounds*

Squat jumps, skater's lunges, chin-ups, push-ups

*Workout 3 – Three rounds; 21, 15, 9 reps*

Walking lunges, pull-ups, burpees, side lunges

# Conclusion and What Comes Next

First of all, congratulations once again on buying this book! It was the important first step in applying more effective exercise techniques to your daily workout routine.

Now that you have completed this book you probably have a lot more knowledge about bodyweight training that you had before. I've laid out the benefits, so you understand by now that bodyweight training is superior to every other exercise regime!

As for what comes next, just remember that starting this workout routine won you half the battle. Now you have to make sure that you keep following this routine for as long as possible.

Starting this exercise routine was hard enough, but unless you keep at it and make sure that the exercises described in this book become a part of your everyday life, you are not going to experience any major benefits.

Once again I would like to thank you for buying this book, and wish you good luck on your journey to a better body!